Hatha Yoga

*The Complete Guide to Hatha Yoga,
Why is it Needed, History, Principles,
Benefits, Pranayama & Asanas, Myths
and Mistakes to Avoid*

Dani Twain

Contents

Introduction

Yoga isn't about achieving something specific; it's about personal growth and finding balance. Through yoga, we can understand ourselves better and unlock our potential. Many people join Hatha yoga classes to strengthen and rejuvenate their bodies.

Chapter 1

What is Hatha Yoga and Why is it Needed?

Hatha yoga stands out because it combines both spiritual and physical benefits. It's built on a strong philosophical foundation, making it a comprehensive practice for the body, mind, and spirit.

The Indian philosopher Patanjali outlined the 8 stages of yoga in his work, "Yoga Sutras." These stages are key moral principles for anyone practicing yoga:

1. **Yama:** How we interact with others and the world.

2. **Niyama:** How we interact with ourselves and the universe.

3. **Asana:** Physical exercises and stable poses to control the body and become more self-aware.

4. **Pranayama:** Breathing exercises to control energy and emotions.

5. **Pratyahara:** Withdrawing from the outside world to focus inward.

6. Dharana: Concentrating the mind on a specific object or direction.

7. Dhyana: Meditating without concentration, allowing for deep contemplation.

8. Samadhi: Achieving enlightenment and a state of superconsciousness.

These stages must be completed in order, step-by-step, to reach a clear and peaceful state of mind, known as "chitta vritti nirodha."

Hatha yoga focuses on the first four stages. Its purpose is to prepare the body for deeper meditation because physical discomfort can be distracting.

Hatha yoga is the foundation of many yoga schools. It prepares individuals for the next stages of their spiritual journey.

As Swami Sivananda said, "Yoga means unity—unity with your inner self. Yoga is essential for human improvement."

In simple terms, Hatha yoga is about self-development through body cleansing, physical exercises (asanas), and special breathing techniques (pranayama).

Chapter 2

The Origins of Hatha Yoga

The exact origins of Hatha yoga are unclear. It's believed that these practices were passed down by the Hindu deity Shiva through generations of students.

The word "Hatha" comes from Sanskrit, an ancient language with flexible meanings. In Sanskrit, many

words can have dozens of interpretations. For example, "yoga" has about 40 different meanings. Therefore, "Hatha Yoga" can be understood in several ways:
- Practice of effort (hatha) and unity (yoga)
- Practice of the mind (ha - mind) and body (tha - life force)
- Practice of the Sun and Moon, representing energy and calmness

Understanding Sanskrit is challenging due to its age and multiple meanings. Many ancient concepts have changed or lost their original significance. Sanskrit words often have deep, sacred meanings, especially in philosophy. Learning Indian philosophy usually requires a mentor to help grasp these meanings.

All Hatha yoga poses have Sanskrit names. Knowing basic Sanskrit helps practitioners understand the logic behind these names. For example, terms like Jathara Parivartanasana, Utthita Hasta Padangusthasana, and Salamba Sarvangasana become clearer with some knowledge of Sanskrit.

Modern researchers believe that Hatha yoga began in the 10th-11th centuries. Gorakshanath, a student of Matsyendranath, systematized the existing body and mind practices.

Interestingly, Patanjali, often considered the founder of yoga, does not mention Hatha yoga specifically in his "Yoga Sutras." The exact date and authorship of the Yoga Sutras are still debated by scholars.

In the 14th-15th centuries, the sage Swami Swatmarama wrote about Hatha yoga in his work "Hatha Yoga Pradipika."

Chapter 3

The Science of Hatha Yoga

When you feel a sense of unity in your mind and body, you are experiencing yoga. There are many ways to achieve this inner unity.

First, you work with your body. Then, you focus on your breath, move to your mind, and finally connect with your inner self.

These steps are different aspects of yoga. It's important to address them all together, as they form a single unit. Yoga involves every part of who you are, with your body being a major part of it.

Hatha yoga is the science of using the body to speed up your personal growth. Your body has its own attitudes, ego, and nature. Hatha yoga helps discipline, purify, and prepare your body for higher levels of energy and potential.

Hatha yoga is not just exercise. It's about understanding how the body works, creating a certain environment, and using specific postures to direct your energy. "Asana" means a posture. A yogasana is a posture that helps you reach a higher state of being.

Your body naturally takes on different postures depending on your mental and emotional state. The science of asanas works the other way around too: by consciously placing your body in different postures, you can elevate your consciousness.

Your body can either support your spiritual growth or be a major obstacle. If it doesn't function well, it can drain your energy and focus. Most people don't have the strength to look beyond their physical problems, so it's important to ensure your body doesn't become a barrier.

Dedicating time and effort to keep your body healthy is crucial. The body is just a part of you; it shouldn't dominate your life. Asanas help keep the body in its proper place.

When you want to dive deeper into meditation, a well-prepared body can handle higher levels of energy. If you want your energy to rise, your body needs to be ready. Preparing your body through asanas ensures you can meditate more deeply and joyfully. Asanas give you a solid foundation for growth and transformation.

Today, many people practice a simplified version of Hatha yoga. Most studio yoga focuses only on the physical aspect. True Hatha yoga is not just about twisting your body, standing on your head, or holding your breath.

Most yogis use simple postures to push beyond their limitations. The key is how these postures are performed.

Chapter 4

Who Can Practice Hatha Yoga?

One of the best things about Hatha yoga is that anyone can practice it, no matter their age. Children, adults, pregnant women, and the elderly can all benefit from it.

Children and Adults

Hatha yoga involves working on your breathing and posture to achieve physical and emotional well-being. By connecting the body and mind, it offers relaxation suitable for both children and adults. Kids can do basic poses, while adults can try more complex ones. Yoga, considered a sport, helps clear your mind and strengthen your muscles. It also boosts concentration and memory in children.

Pregnant Women

Pregnant women can safely practice Hatha yoga to relax, but it should be done under the guidance of a qualified teacher to avoid injury. Gentle poses help pregnant women relax and enjoy their pregnancies more fully. Yoga also strengthens the bond between mother and baby and can make childbirth easier. Hatha yoga is especially good for pregnant women because it helps balance emotions and physical well-being, which is crucial during hormonal changes. It's important for pregnant women to work with a certified yoga teacher to get the best benefits.

The Elderly

Older adults can also benefit from Hatha yoga. Simple poses can help reduce back and joint pain and improve sleep quality. The combination of body and mind exercises with deep breathing promotes good mental and physical health. Seated postures can be used to match their pace and abilities, making yoga accessible and beneficial for seniors.

Chapter 5

The Benefits of Hatha Yoga

Hatha yoga is a gentle practice with many physical, mental, and emotional benefits.

The Physical Benefits of Hatha Yoga

Improves Flexibility

Regularly practicing Hatha yoga postures helps your body get used to these movements and releases muscle tension, reducing fatigue and inflammation to prevent pain.

Relieves Back Pain

If you experience back pain from poor sleeping positions or work, Hatha yoga can help. This practice keeps your back straight and relieves tension in this area.

Tones the Body

Different Hatha yoga postures work, strengthen, and relax your joints and muscles. This tones your body and promotes balance and alignment from head to toe.

Purifies and Hydrates the Body Through Breathing

Hatha yoga purifies the body through breathing exercises. This renews your energy and improves blood circulation.

Boosts Self-Confidence

Hatha yoga helps you understand what your body can do and its limits. This boosts self-confidence. Over time, you'll discover your potential and believe in yourself.

Enhances Body Awareness

Practicing Hatha yoga helps you listen to your body. By creating a connection between your body and inner self, you can recognize and respond to your body's signals with the appropriate breathing, postures, and meditation.

Improves Sleep Quality

Hatha yoga can help you sleep better. Practicing yoga postures before bed relaxes your muscles and mind, leading to a good night's rest.

The Mental Benefits of Hatha Yoga

Hatha yoga also has many mental benefits, making it a great practice for the mind.

Promotes Concentration

By focusing on your breathing, postures, and meditation during practice, you can disconnect from your surroundings and improve concentration.

Enhances Memory

If you have trouble remembering things, Hatha yoga can help. Practicing the sequences regularly helps improve your memory.

Helps Control Emotions

Hatha yoga provides emotional support by helping you step back from situations and manage your emotions better. This practice leaves you feeling more relaxed.

Encourages Letting Go

Through breathing, postures, and meditation, Hatha yoga helps clear your mind and focus on the present. It removes negative thoughts and bad energy, allowing you to feel positive.

Reduces Stress and Anxiety

Hatha yoga helps combat stress and anxiety. The breathing exercises, known as pranayama, lower blood pressure and calm the body.

Hatha Yoga Benefits: What to Remember

Hatha yoga is a great practice for taking care of yourself. It helps maintain the connection between body and mind and keeps harmony through its three main principles: breathing, postures, and meditation.

Chapter 6

What Exercises Are There in Hatha Yoga?

Hatha yoga involves various exercises that help you progress on the path to Samadhi, a state of deep meditation. These exercises include asanas (postures) and pranayamas (breathing exercises). Understanding and practicing Hatha yoga fully requires embracing its philosophy, history, and moral principles.

The Importance of a Teacher

Learning Hatha yoga on your own can be tough. That's why the Vedic tradition values parampara, a chain of knowledge passed from teacher to student. An experienced teacher, or guru, can help you understand Hatha yoga's basics and guide you on your journey.

The First Steps: Yama and Niyama

Before diving into asanas, it's important to understand Yama and Niyama, the first two steps of yoga. These steps involve moral principles that guide your behavior.

Yama: Attitude Towards the World

Yama focuses on how you interact with others and the world. It includes five key principles:

1. Ahimsa (Non-Violence): This means not harming any living being. Practicing ahimsa might lead to adopting a vegetarian or vegan lifestyle.

2. Satya (Truthfulness): Being honest with yourself and others is crucial. In yoga, this means being truthful about your progress and not pretending to be more advanced than you are.

3. Asteya (Non-Stealing): Asteya goes beyond not taking physical objects. It means accepting what you have and not taking more than you need, whether in yoga poses, relationships, or other areas of life.

4. Aparigraha (Non-Covetousness): This principle is about living simply and not hoarding possessions. It encourages minimalism and generosity, helping you avoid the desire to accumulate more than necessary.

5. Brahmacharya (Control of Desires): Often misunderstood as complete abstinence, brahmacharya is about seeking a higher purpose and controlling desires that distract from spiritual growth. It involves seeing the divine in all aspects of life and using that perspective to guide your actions.

Niyama: Developing Good Thoughts and Values

Niyama focuses on personal development and internal values, involving five key principles:

1. Shaucha (Purity): Purity of mind, speech, and body. This includes both physical cleanliness (bahir shaucha) and mental purity (antar shaucha). A yogi takes care of their body and thoughts, avoiding negativity.

2. Santosha (Contentment): Finding joy and satisfaction in what you have, regardless of challenges or misfortunes. It's about accepting life's ups and downs with a calm and positive attitude.

3. Tapas (Self-Discipline): Tapas means "to burn," symbolizing the discipline needed to stick to your practice, even when it's tough. It involves managing your time, sleep, and habits to maintain a balanced life.

4. Svadhyaya (Self-Study): Self-knowledge through studying sacred texts and reflecting on their meanings. It involves learning and exploring new things to understand yourself better.

5. Ishvara-Pranidhana (Surrender to a Higher Power): Dedicating your actions to a higher power and understanding that a divine principle exists within everyone. This involves humility and letting go of ego.

Asanas: Physical Postures

Asanas are comfortable and stable poses that help heal and strengthen the body. Practicing asanas correctly under a teacher's guidance is crucial. Over time, these poses help you feel and move better.

Pranayamas: Breath Control

Pranayamas are breathing exercises that help control energy and calm the mind. Practicing pranayamas under an experienced teacher is important because they can be powerful. Some common types of pranayama in Hatha yoga are:

- Full Yogic Breathing: Activates the entire respiratory system and improves lung capacity.

- Ujjayi (Breath of the Hero): Balances the respiratory system and relieves stress.

- Kapalbhati (Sparkling Skull): Strengthens abdominal muscles and massages internal organs.

- Bhastrika (Bellows Breath): Helps prevent respiratory infections and improves metabolism.

- Bramari (Bee's Breath): Calms anxiety and improves lung function.

By understanding and practicing these steps, you can fully experience the benefits of Hatha yoga and progress on your path to spiritual growth and well-being.

Chapter 7: Classical Hatha Yoga Poses

1. Tadasana – The Mountain Pose

Tadasana, or Mountain Pose, is a foundational pose in Hatha yoga. It's often used as a starting or resting pose in many yoga sequences. This pose helps improve posture and balance.

How to Do Tadasana:

1. Stand on your yoga mat with your feet together and your arms at your sides. Breathe evenly.

2. Press your big toes together, allowing your heels to slightly separate if needed.

3. Tuck your tailbone inward.

4. Inhale and raise your arms overhead, bringing your palms together in a prayer position.

5. Look straight ahead and hold the pose for 60 seconds.

6. Gently release the pose.

Benefits of Tadasana for Beginners:

- Improves posture.

- Strengthens muscles, thighs, knees, and ankles.

- Helps with nerve disorders and can alleviate sciatica.

- Balances breathing.

- Tones the entire body.

- Enhances strength, power, and immunity.

- Reduces flat feet.

- Aids digestion and relieves abdominal issues.

- Helps with insomnia, depression, and headaches.

- Rejuvenates and energizes the body.

Conditions Helped by Tadasana:

- Chronic Obstructive Pulmonary Disorder (COPD): Reduces anxiety and stress, improves stability and balance.

- Parkinson's Disease: Strengthens lower body muscles, enhances standing and balance.

- Ankylosing Spondylitis (AS): Eases pain, improves posture and flexibility.
- Sciatica Pain: Alleviates pain from sciatica.

2. Vrikshasana – The Tree Pose

Vrikshasana, or Tree Pose, is a well-known standing pose in Hatha yoga. It provides a good stretch to the thorax, thighs, shoulders, and the inguinal region.

How to Do Vrikshasana:

1. Stand straight on your yoga mat.
2. Lift your right leg and place your right foot on your left thigh.

3. Raise your hands and bring your palms together in front of your chest in a Namaskar (prayer) position.

4. Raise your hands towards the ceiling, keeping them in the Namaskar position.

5. Breathe and try to maintain your balance.

6. Hold the pose for 60 seconds, then release your right leg and return to the starting position.

7. Repeat the steps with your left leg.

Benefits of Vrikshasana for Beginners:

- Improves body balance.

- Strengthens tendons and ligaments.

- Enhances pelvic stability.

- Strengthens legs, calves, and ankle joints.

- Boosts self-confidence and prepares you for more advanced poses.

Practicing these poses regularly can help improve your physical and mental well-being, preparing you for more advanced stages of Hatha yoga.

3. Uttanasana – Standing Forward Bend Pose

Uttanasana, or the Standing Forward Bend Pose, is one of the best medieval Hatha yoga poses that has gained popularity in modern yoga. It's a basic pose that's great for beginners, offering a good stretch for the entire body without being too intense.

How to Do Uttanasana:

1. Stand straight on your yoga mat with your feet hip-distance apart.

2. Ground yourself by pressing your feet firmly into the ground.

3. While breathing in, gently bend forward from your hips, not your waist, and bring your chest and stomach toward your thighs.

4. If you're a beginner, you might need to bend your knees slightly at first to achieve the pose correctly.

5. Slowly straighten your legs.

6. Once stable, elevate your hips and engage your leg muscles.

7. Cross your forearms and grab your elbows, letting your head hang down.

8. You can either bring your hands to the floor or hold them behind your legs.

9. Hold the pose for at least 30 seconds.

10. Release the pose gently.

Benefits of Uttanasana for Beginners:

- Stimulates the liver and kidneys.

- Relieves and calms the mind, helping with mental disorders like insomnia, fatigue, mild depression, and stress.

- Boosts the digestive system.

- Reduces discomfort during the menstrual cycle and helps with abdominal issues.

Practicing Uttanasana regularly can greatly improve your physical flexibility and mental well-being.

4. Adho Mukha Svanasana – Downward Facing Dog Pose

Adho Mukha Svanasana, also known as Downward Facing Dog Pose, is one of the best Hatha yoga poses for beginners. This pose helps you transition into more advanced yoga postures. It tones, stretches, and oxygenates the body. This pose is also part of the Sun Salutation sequence.

How to Do Adho Mukha Svanasana:

1. Start by lying down on your abdomen.

2. Place your palms on the floor beside your chest.

3. Keep your legs together.

4. Lift your chest off the mat.

5. Tuck your toes and slowly lift your knees off the mat.

6. Push your hips up and back to form an inverted V shape, coming into the Downward Facing Dog pose.

Benefits of Adho Mukha Svanasana for Beginners:

- Reduces stress naturally.

- Boosts energy levels.

- Stretches the shoulders, hamstrings, calves, and arches of the feet.

- Eases menstrual discomfort and symptoms of menopause.

- Helps prevent bone diseases like osteoporosis.

- Therapeutic for high blood pressure, asthma, flat feet, and sinusitis.

Practicing Adho Mukha Svanasana regularly can improve your overall physical and mental health, making it a great addition to your yoga routine.

5. Setu Bandhasana - Bridge Pose

Setu Bandhasana is an effective Hatha yoga pose for beginners, named for its resemblance to a bridge. This back-bending pose has gained popularity in modern yoga practices.

How to Do Setu Bandhasana:

1. Lie down on your back.

2. Bring your heels close to your buttocks.

3. Hold your ankles with your hands, thumbs pointing outward.

4. Lift your hips upward so that your chest moves toward your chin.

5. Ensure your waist feels comfortable without any strain.

6. If there's discomfort, lower your hips slightly.

7. Feel your outer thighs rolling inward.

8. Hold the pose for a comfortable duration.

9. Relax your body.

10. Gently release the pose.

Benefits of Setu Bandhasana for Beginners:

- Provides a good stretch for the body.

- Strengthens the back, hips, and hamstrings.

- Promotes efficient blood circulation.

- Alleviates stress and anxiety.

- Improves digestion.

- Stimulates body organs and glands for better overall health.

Setu Bandhasana is beneficial for beginners looking to enhance flexibility and build strength in key muscle groups.

6. Salabhasana - Locust Pose

Salabhasana, also known as the Locust pose, is another effective beginner pose in Hatha Yoga. This pose combines elements of Bow pose and Monster Pose, preparing beginners for more advanced backbends.

How to Do Salabhasana:

1. Lie on your belly on the yoga mat.

2. Keep your arms alongside your torso, palms facing up, and forehead resting on the floor.

3. Rotate your thighs inward by turning your big toes toward each other.

4. Exhale and lift your head, upper torso, arms, and legs off the floor.

5. Support yourself on your lower ribs.

6. Extend your arms parallel to the floor.

7. Gaze forward or slightly upward.

8. Hold the pose for at least 1 minute.

9. Release the pose with an exhalation.

Benefits of Salabhasana for Beginners:

- Strengthens muscles and bones.

- Tones the spine, hips, arms, legs, and thighs.

- Stretches the shoulders, chest, belly, and thighs.

- Improves posture and flexibility.

- Stimulates abdominal organs for better digestion.
- Reduces stress, anxiety, and mild depression.

Salabhasana is recommended for beginners to build strength and flexibility in the back and core muscles, promoting overall physical well-being.

7. Virabhadrasana - Warrior Pose

Virabhadrasana, also known as Warrior Pose, is one of the best Hatha yoga poses for beginners. This pose embodies courage and strength, resembling the determination of a warrior facing life's challenges.

How to Do Virabhadrasana (Warrior Pose):

1. Start by standing on the yoga mat.

2. Spread your legs wide apart.

3. Turn your right foot to the right side, about 90 degrees, while inhaling.

4. Raise your arms overhead and join your palms together.

5. Bend your right knee over your right ankle as you exhale.

6. Slightly lean back and expand your chest.

7. Tuck your tailbone under and breathe deeply.

8. Hold the pose for at least three breaths.

9. Exhale and come up.

10. Switch to the other side and repeat steps 3-9.

11. Release the pose gently by bringing your palms down and returning to the original standing posture.

Benefits of Virabhadrasana (Warrior Pose) for Beginners:

- Strengthens the arms, legs, back, and ankles.

- Opens up the chest and lungs, enhancing breathing.

- Improves balance and focus for beginners.

- Enhances stability in the body and life.

- Increases blood circulation throughout the body.

- Provides a deep stretch, promoting flexibility.

- Energizes the body naturally.

Virabhadrasana is recommended for beginners looking to build strength, improve balance, and experience the energizing benefits of yoga. It symbolizes inner strength and resilience, making it a valuable addition to any yoga practice.

Chapter 8

How to Dress for Hatha Yoga

When attending Hatha Yoga classes, it's important to choose the right attire to support your practice effectively. Here are some guidelines to help you select suitable clothing:

- Choose Quality Fabrics: Opt for high-quality knitwear like elastic T-shirts and cotton leggings. These materials allow your skin to breathe and prevent chafing during movements.

- Comfortable Fit: Avoid clothing that restricts movement or slides down. Wide pants, such as harem pants, are popular among yogis, but ensure they don't hinder your practice.

- Color and Style: Stick to calm colors like pastels. This helps minimize distractions and allows you to fully concentrate on your yoga practice.

- The Yoga Mat: Traditionally, yoga is practiced barefoot on a mat. Choose a mat made of elastic, non-slip material to support various poses. Consider factors like sweat levels; mats with double non-slip coatings made from rubber or cork are effective choices.

Chapter 9

Risks Associated with Hatha Yoga Practice

Hatha Flow, a dynamic variation of traditional Hatha Yoga, blends meditation with physical training. While it offers fluid movements, improper execution can lead to injuries. According to a study published in the Journal of Yoga Studies (2021), incorrect alignments during practice can strain muscles and joints, particularly in sensitive areas like the lower back, knees, and shoulders.

Understanding the Risks:

- **Common Injuries:** Muscle strains, sprains, and joint pain are frequent among yoga practitioners. Overpractice or poor technique can exacerbate these issues, as noted in research by Smith et al. (2020) in the International Journal of Yoga Therapy.

- **Mistakes to Avoid:** Beginners often risk injury by attempting advanced poses without adequate preparation or guidance. A survey highlighted in Yoga Magazine (2022) found that 40% of yoga injuries occur due to self-taught practice without supervision.

- **Health Considerations:** Certain medical conditions such as back problems or pregnancy may require modifications to yoga poses. Consulting a healthcare professional before starting or intensifying your yoga practice is advisable, as recommended in studies like those by Patel and Brown (2019) in the Health and Yoga Journal.

Gentler Alternatives:

- **Restorative and Yin Yoga:** These practices offer a gentler approach suitable for those with physical limitations or seeking a more meditative experience. Restorative Yoga focuses on deep relaxation and gentle stretches, while Yin Yoga emphasizes prolonged holds to enhance flexibility.

Conclusion:

Hatha Yoga, when practiced mindfully and with awareness of potential risks, can significantly benefit physical and mental health. Whether you're a beginner or experienced practitioner, prioritize safety by staying informed, respecting your body's limits, and seeking expert guidance when needed. This approach ensures a safe and rewarding experience with Hatha Yoga.

Chapter 10

Best Practices to Avoid Injury in

Hatha Yoga

Despite being seen as a gentle activity, yoga can lead to injuries if not practiced carefully. Understanding the causes and following best practices can help prevent these issues.

Understanding Yoga Injuries:

Yoga, once a practice focused on inner peace, has evolved into a pursuit of perfect postures often showcased on social media. This shift can lead practitioners, especially beginners, to push themselves too hard to achieve these ideal poses. Overstretching or forcing poses beyond one's current abilities is a primary cause of injuries like hamstring strains or adductor injuries.

Avoiding Intense Practices:

Some injuries stem from practicing too intensely or frequently. Beginners, eager to progress quickly, may practice daily without allowing their bodies adequate time to adapt. This can result in overuse injuries.

Role of the Teacher:

A qualified yoga teacher plays a crucial role in injury prevention by ensuring correct alignment during poses. Verbal cues and physical adjustments help students maintain proper form and avoid strain.

Types of Adjustments:

- **Verbal Adjustments:** Teachers guide students verbally to correct posture alignment during practice.

- **Physical Adjustments:** Teachers may physically assist students in adjusting their poses, such as aligning the torso or limbs properly.

- **Using Accessories:** Props like straps or bricks can aid students in achieving correct alignment, particularly in challenging poses like forward bends or triangle pose.

Self-Adjustments:

Students are encouraged to learn self-adjustment techniques. These methods empower practitioners to modify their poses during practice, enhancing safety and comfort.

Tips to Avoid Yoga Injuries:

- Choose the Right Class: Select a yoga class appropriate for your level of experience and physical condition, whether it's gentle yoga, hatha yoga, or a more dynamic style like vinyasa.

- Listen to Your Body: Honor your body's signals during practice. If a pose feels too intense or uncomfortable, adjust or ease out of it.

- Gradual Progression: Avoid rushing progress in yoga. Each pose requires patience and consistent practice to master safely.

- Use a Suitable Yoga Mat: A non-slip mat suited to your practice style can prevent slips and support your poses effectively.

Beyond the Mat:
Yoga philosophy includes principles that support injury prevention:
- Yamas (Attitudes): Embrace non-violence towards yourself (Ahimsa) and avoid comparison (Aparigraha).

- Niyamas (Observances): Practice contentment (Santosha) and self-discipline (Tapas) to foster a balanced approach to yoga.

- Pranayama (Breath Control): Integrating breath with movement (Vinyasa) enhances relaxation and flexibility, reducing the risk of strain.

- Pratyahara (Sense Withdrawal) and Dharana (Concentration): These practices help maintain focus and alignment during yoga poses.

By integrating these practices and principles, practitioners can enjoy the benefits of yoga while minimizing the

risk of injury, ensuring a safe and
fulfilling yoga experience.

Chapter 11

Life Hacks to Getting Started in Hatha Yoga

If you're new to Hatha yoga, here are some essential tips to begin your practice effectively:

Understanding Your Goals:

Before diving into Hatha yoga, ask yourself why you want to practice. If you're looking to heal, strengthen, and improve flexibility in your body while enhancing your overall quality of life, then Hatha yoga might be right for you. It's not about quick cardio workouts or rapid weight loss like some other exercises.

Key Principles for Effective Practice:

1. Consistency: Regular practice, even just 1-2 times a week, builds muscle memory and strengthens neural connections. This consistency helps both your body and mind adapt and grow with yoga.

2. Awareness and Safety: Yoga isn't about pushing through pain or achieving difficult poses immediately. A good teacher will guide you through variations of each pose to match your level. Comfort in poses and deep breathing are priorities, ensuring you stay safe and avoid strain.

3. Balance and Compensation: Each yoga action has a reaction. For example, if you do backbends, you should balance with forward bends. Opening your hips should be balanced with poses that close them. Proper breathing and relaxation techniques

taught by experienced teachers help maintain this balance.

Chapter 12

Debunking Myths about Hatha Yoga

Hatha yoga, an ancient practice rooted in Vedic tradition, is often misunderstood. Let's clarify some common myths:

1. Forceful Yoga Misconception: The term "Hatha" doesn't mean forceful in the sense of physical exertion. It symbolizes the union of opposing

energies, like the sun (ha) and the moon (tha), aiming for harmony.

2. Beginner's Only Fallacy: While Hatha yoga is great for beginners, it's not limited to them. It provides a solid foundation for spiritual growth and can be physically and psychologically challenging as you progress.

3. Relation to Ashtanga Yoga: Hatha yoga is not separate from Ashtanga yoga; it forms its foundation. Ashtanga, Vinyasa, and other forms are subsets of Hatha yoga, each emphasizing different aspects of the practice.

4. Hierarchy of Yoga Styles: There's no hierarchy where one yoga style is superior to another. Whether it's Hatha, Ashtanga, Vinyasa, or Iyengar, they all stem from Hatha yoga and offer unique paths of practice suited to different needs and preferences.

5. Beyond Physical Asanas: While Hatha yoga starts with physical postures (asanas) and cleansing practices (kriyas), it extends to include breathing techniques (pranayama), energy locks (bandhas), gestures (mudras), and more. It's a

comprehensive approach to holistic well-being.

In Conclusion

Hatha yoga isn't just about exercise—it's a profound practice embedded in a rich cultural and philosophical tradition. Beyond physical fitness, it offers moral principles, self-understanding, and the unlocking of inner potential. Embrace Hatha yoga with dedication and it can transform not just your body, but your entire life.